Copyright © 2019 Shannon Marie.

All rights reserved. This book or any portion thereof may not be reproduced or used in any manner whatsoever without the express written permission of the publisher except for the use of brief quotations in a book review.

First printing, 2019.

10qaa Publishing

14800 Duffy Road

Hinckley, IL 60520

www.10qaa.com

10 Questions People Ask Me About Lyme Disease

Asked- ☑
&
Answered- ☑

Table of Contents

Introduction P. 5

#1 Can people die from Lyme disease? P.15

#2 If I have Lyme and become pregnant could the disease be passed in utero? P.29

#3 Is there anything I can do to be certain not to get Lyme? P.37

#4 Is it necessary to maintain a strict diet while fighting Lyme? P.47

#5 Does Lyme disease come from ticks alone? P.57

#6 What is a predator to ticks? P.63

#7 What is a co-infection? P.69

#8 You appear to be fine on the outside, so why aren't you working? P.79

#9 What one piece of advice would you offer to those still in the fight against Lyme? P.87

#10 Do you wish you never went for that hike? P.93

Conclusion P.97

For Further Study P.101

About the Author P.103

Introduction

Lyme became a big part of my life prior to being diagnosed. For seven years, I lived with Lyme without knowing what was happening to my body. I began to lose abilities and experience a wide range of completely unrelated symptoms.

First, for me, my legs began to burn from the knee down so badly I would basically lay awake scratching them in hopes I would rip my skin off. Breathing was difficult at times as well; I remember being in a store with my youngest child when all the sudden it was as if I was breathing through a tiny straw; I simply sat down in the aisle having no idea what was happening. I would make my way from Dr. to Dr. sharing these, what can be seen as completely unrelated symptoms, in hopes someone could tell me what was happening to me.

Lyme disease maintains its mysteriousness when given opportunity to multiply within the human body. I did not know I had Lyme when I actually contracted it; I barely even knew what Lyme was. I simply thought we had a nice little family hike and then soon thereafter I had some nasty flu. I didn't heed the warning from my body which is why knowledge is so powerful.

Throughout the next seven years, new symptoms were emerging left and right. Now, because Lyme had plenty of time to play around in my body, I began to deal with more than the initial infection. Lyme disease can include co-infections as well which will take the opportunity to attack any and all systems within the body. Yes, it is optimal to treat Lyme when one first recognizes the bullseye rash, however, and unfortunately, the majority of those stricken do not see the rash.

I remember that hike. I remember how hot it was outside while my husband found that snake and the kids were mesmerized. I thought I was simply taking a walk with my family, all the while, my life was about to take a drastic turn. Life, after all, can do that. We can be going along to get along and then in an instant, life will never be the same. How many people have been affected by Lyme and how many are affected by walking this battle with a family member? I did not know slicing pizza was a privilege until I lost it. I did not know I would have to pray before entering the grocery store on several occasions, sometimes never making it inside the door because I was too shaky to walk a straight line. I was never aware of what it felt like to struggle to simply breathe. I certainly never knew I would desire the end to simply stop living through such physical pain.

"But you have children, Shannon, how could you desire the end when they need you?"

My children were not living a typical life, in fact, my children were subjected to just as much darkness as I was, maybe even more. It is hard to desire to be there for your family and yet, you simply cannot. It is hard, yes, to watch life around you all the while, you cannot wait to be asleep as that is your only escape from the brutal world of Lyme disease and the harshness behind each co-infection. I would lie awake crying hoping for the end because I became so weary of what my children had already seen and witnessed. However, my children are the very reason I would continue to choose to fight.

Going into this battle, there's an understanding that it will take time to win. That can be hard, extremely hard, when the present day leaves us keeled over. We desire to be well right now and that is human nature. How can we take the day to day and truthfully second by second at times fighting this war and search for the positive? Lyme came into my life and stole much yet left me with no other option but to open my eyes to the World. Now, I cannot walk through a grocery store without wondering if anyone in there is struggling to shop, and praying they can successfully endure the checkout process.

I lived years behind my sunglasses, indoors and out, due to such sensitivities. The looks, yes I saw them but soon you simply do not care. After all, if I didn't head out in a hat or glasses, I would have missed much of my children's events. Who knew? Who knew that life would become simply doing all I could to not pass out. Pass out, I did. Five grand mal seizures later and yet, still here, still breathing.

Lyme comes to overtake, steal, and destroy. It did. It has. Yet, part of the journey is trying desperately to find any little positive victory. The fight is long and hard. Support can seem dismal and at times, even antagonizing. Where do we go for help? I tried to find help through so many Doctors only to be treated with such a lack of understanding or compassion. I tried to explain myself to just about anybody in hopes that they would understand. Then we break. We cannot continue to be so brave; it is essential to have moments of despair because it is truly healing to get it all out. So many things can affect our healing and I truly believe stuffing emotions deep down inside will hinder our necessary peace to fight back and win.

Yes, treatment helps but we are our best defense to taking a multifaceted approach to healing. A whole body detox to fight back. Holding back forgiveness and pretending to have it all under control without admitting we need help are two areas of healing the Lord brought to my heart. If we want to be truly healed; we must be willing to open doors we have maybe had shut for years, even decades.

Lyme disease rips, tears, and breaks families apart. My family tore apart easily and headed straight for the lovely Court system. Three wonderful children, Lyme disease, impending divorce, brain surgery, and simply taking one day at a time and that was life; that was life for years. There is positive if we look for it. My PICC line was to be inserted and the RN was teaching me how to administer my own treatment without moving that line.

I was not looking forward to that at all for a few reasons. Medication will for sure head in and kill the bad guys, however, it will also take the good guys with him. I knew I had to endure this but the mental game of thinking about my immune system being hit hard was very difficult to deal with. Just another phase, I would tell myself, and then we would spend months detoxing. There I was, she had arrived, and I was all set to get that PICC line inserted, "Turn your head to the left; here we go." I turned my head and said, "God..." I had nothing. Then, without thought, "Hold me help me," came to heart and that tiny prayer carried me through years of my fight with Lyme.

There was the positive, I heard directly from the Lord in that hospital room. He was there. I was not alone. The Lord knew what I had been through and He knows where I am headed and He wants to be there every step of the way. I didn't know that before. I mean I might have known that from hearing it preached that God is with you always. I had heard it, sure, and I guess I believed it, sure, but now I lived it. There is a difference. God was now, in that hospital room, showing Himself to me, His daughter.

What I had heard was true, but I held that like religion. I believed it but I lived my life going about it day by day not really knowing there was anything more beyond the religion of Jesus Christ. I learned as He allowed this suffering in my life, that He was desperately pursuing me in hopes to have a relationship. Relationship is different from religion. In my religion, I agreed with what I learned but in a relationship, I found a God who loves me. I found a God willing to speak to me daily and who had a desire to go each and every step with me. I found that I needed Him in my life, not just that I believed He existed but that I knew I needed His existence in every single day of my life. I did not know that before my battle through the dark valley with Lyme.

Why does God allow suffering? A question I dare say we all have faced at some point. The easy answer is the Bible declares we will suffer and after all, He did for us so why should we just skate through. Personally, it was through suffering that I found His love for me; through Lyme, I found Christ's love for me to be true and everlasting. God will do what He can to pursue His children because He loves. What a trip it has been and what a journey that we are still on. All along the tears, hanging by not a thread but after the thread is already splitting; hanging by the last split line and ready to quit, the screams, the pain, the heartbreak, the unforeseen hurdles along the way; Lyme will do its very best to take control of your life, your family, your finances, your faith and sadly for many, your future.

I seek to educate, yes, but I also seek to build warriors out of all precious Lyme fighters. Laying in that bed in Tennessee, unable to move much, looking out that window and thinking okay Lord, I'm ready to come home. Wow, was I given such grace that day. Thank God the Lord has taken me on this journey to finding faith. I can only imagine, humorously the Lord's reaction when I said those words, "Girl, you may feel ready but you ain't coming to My home!" Ok, God does not talk like that but it's the point I'm trying to drive home.

The road is long and scary at times; quitting looks really good at times and yet, come win the battle with me. Many have asked, allow me to now give an answer to ten questions people have asked me about Lyme disease.

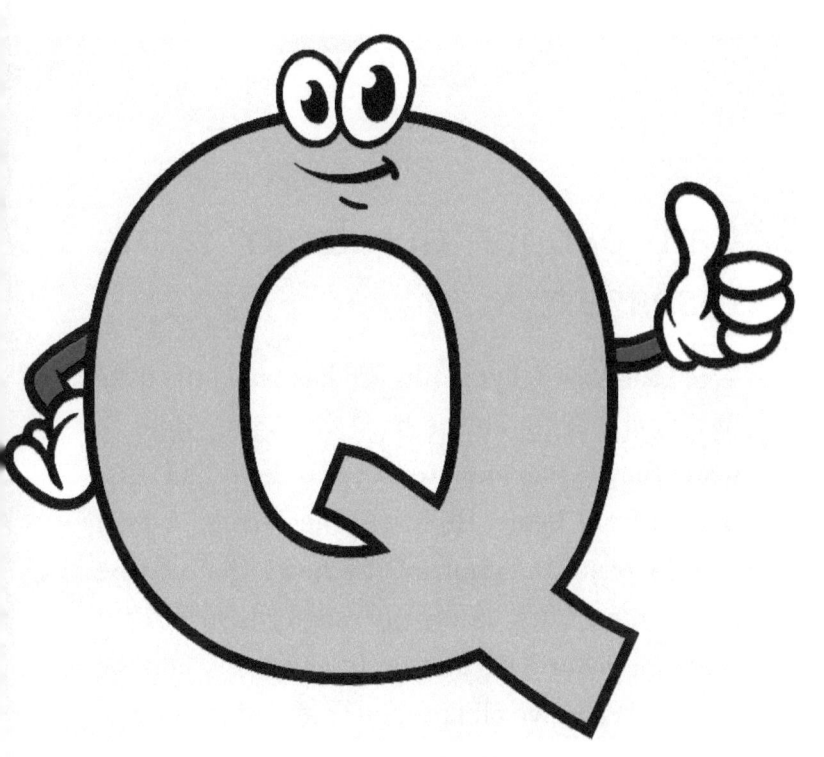

#1

Can people die from Lyme disease?

Sadly, yes. Lyme disease has taken the lives of many; it truly hit me hard during my fight to hear that a seventeen-year-old boy had just passed from Lyme. He had Lyme carditis, which is a bacterial infection of the heart that can be fatal. When I first knew my diagnosis in 2014, I was not aware of the community I would be joining. When we all face any trial in this life, one of the blessings in the midst is who we now understand and who can understand us. Allow me to explain.

I walked around with Lyme disease since 2007 but did not realize what was taking over my mind and body for seven years. The minute I heard, "Sorry, you have late-stage chronic Lyme disease," I immediately became a part of a new family. Now, I yearned to understand Lyme and its intricacies; I also began to realize I was not the only one who walked this long, dark and truly frightening road. There was a peace in the diagnosis that I had never had in those seven lonely years, waiting for anyone to say, "I get it." For the first time in a long time, what I was saying now made sense.

Sadly, in the difficulty of living Lyme life amidst others who cannot understand or do not even try to, Lyme can bring on devastating depression. While the Lyme can cause death itself, the difficult journey is also causing a very real issue with suicide in the Lyme community. This breaks my heart personally because I understand very well how broken one can become and just how hopeless this disease can feel. I would be lying to you if I did not admit taking my life did not come into my mind several times throughout my Lyme journey.

When I was lying in that bed and watching my three children playing outside and I could not be with them, I wanted it to end. When showering became a chore, and my goal was to not fall out of that tub, I wanted it to end. I would sit at times, up in bed, and watch the cars driving by, thinking to myself, life is real to that person yet, I am simply alive. I exist. I am here. That's about it. Walking my kids to the bus stop became impossible. Dizziness became my normal way of life; I wondered what it would be like to not feel drunk daily? Ironically, I do not drink and yet, I've lived for years feeling drunk.

Lying there in bed, clawing at my legs, genuinely believing if I just ripped off the skin, it wouldn't burn so bad. So yes, truth be told, suicide is very real within our Lyme family; I believe it breaks my heart so deeply because I know just how that precious person felt in that moment. I, too, had those moments. They are not few and far between, they can be daily, even by the minute. I have three children and I know that I have zero credit when it comes to me not succumbing to suicide. By the grace of God, I am still here. I could not and would not have made it as far as I have if I did not get real with Jesus.

Too often, and I am guilty of this myself, we tend to live, "I got this." Even as Christians, we can walk around praising God and yet, never leaving the driver's seat. I have a dear friend, Jill, who has walked this road right alongside me; we would joke how we both can say, "OK Lord, take the wheel why don't YA!" The Lord's looking at us thinking I'll take that wheel when you take your hands off, unbuckle, and get out of My perfect way but I will not remove you as this is a choice you must make. Do we want to trust in ourselves or do we want to trust in God? Seems like a no brainer yet, Shannon tends to jump from the backseat to the wheel again constantly!

Sometimes, I'm grabbing for the wheel and not even knowing it and then I crash and say, "God, what are You doing?!" God didn't do anything because again, I decided I had better control over the situation. We fear. We fear what we cannot see. Here's my reference to Indiana Jones, the scene when Harrison Ford needs to step out and trust that path is going to be there; we struggle in faith when we need to trust the road ahead when we cannot see one foot in front of us. Lord, do you see me when I struggle to breathe from Chlamydia Pneumonia attacking my lungs? Lord, do you care that I am struggling to walk or continue to run into walls from this hellish dizziness? Lord, how am I supposed to take care of my children when I cannot even take care of myself? I wanted the answer; I wanted the whole picture.

Truthfully, I struggled to trust in the Lord with all my heart and stop trying to understand the situation. I didn't want to acknowledge Him, I simply wanted to heal and right now! Submission in suffering during Lyme life was a frightening choice to make. I cried several tears simply laying there looking up at the ceiling. All those nights that I had questions; all those nights that I didn't know how I would face tomorrow. Crying out loud, waking up with night sweats, or never even falling asleep only to see the sun begin to rise. Faint whispering to God, "Are you even here?" Weeks of beginning to pray and having absolutely nothing to say. Like Jacob, I spent years wrestling with God. All the tears, all the questions, all the screams, all the silence, every single emotion I shared with my Lord, it was in these moments, my religion turned into my relationship.

Religion can believe, it can quote, it can easily point the finger, and to all of that I am guilty, yet, it is in a relationship where we find His love, His grace, and it is where we find our hope. Without this hope, again I ache for all my Lyme family that ended their life. I do not judge; I only lament and mourn. Occasionally, I spend time on one of our Lyme memorial sites to simply mourn those in the family of Lyme that has passed. As I scroll, I read different infections causing death (Many of which I too have had), death by grand mal seizure (Of which I have had five) or painful suicide, which I just tear up and well up with compassion (As I too, understand the brokenness).

Yet, I am still here so may God give me a voice to help others with Lyme; I will push forward always remembering every precious life lost. What if you're watching a family member suffer greatly and you are now worried about them? The pressures of life are what put me over the edge; after I sold my car and diamond ring for money, how would I take care of my children? Yes, to simply spend time, sitting with your loved one fighting is very helpful. Being able to listen and do your best to understand what they are going through. Maybe putting time into your own research, calling their Doctors to better understand, even joining a group yourselves through this journey could be helpful. Trying to be cautious with questions as well; during the fight as we are trying to heal, our energy can only be spent on surpassing each treatment. Added pressures can truly add great stress to one trying to beat this disease.

Yes, conversations are good, and communication is necessary, however, try leaving any judging or assuming aside. Do not assume as one is up and showered that they are in a place to seek employment. Lyme kills from the inside; we may look or appear to be fine but in reality, we may be dealing with pain, inflammation issues, gut issues which are very real with Lyme, or the threatening emotional and mental side of this fight. How many have lost a loved one to suicide and thought they never expected that to happen and did not see it coming. Those with Lyme, feeling this depth of sadness, it is necessary to be as open and honest as possible with our families. Our families then need to be willing to hear and best understand where we are.

If you are fighting Lyme alone, please seek counsel, even from a community Church; one call to the Pastor can help set up support around you. Music helped me many a night; just lying there and filling my mind with hope, even if I didn't feel hopeful. Writing a book with my kids, giving my mind something else to focus on, even if we never sold one copy. My parents would randomly bring me Chipotle and to them it was nothing but to me, it was everything in that one day. Dear friends would stop by with groceries or food from our Church's food pantry. A special friend's family even stepped in and drove my daughter to school each day. Trust when I say, even the little things we all can be doing to help as best we can be truly priceless. Writing notes of encouragement; I received some over the years and the encouragement from others can go a long way in fighting one more day.

Lyme community, taking the good from others and remaining grateful while not accepting the bad can become very real. As I say to my children, all you need is one really good friend and you're set. All you need too, is one that you can call and just get it out, is all you need. God is there, yes, always to lament to and even finding a story in the Bible or praying that God lays one on your heart to feel understood. Believe me, the lady who bled for twelve years and finally found her healing, and I have some special connection and hopefully, I'll meet her one day.

Look at David, read the Psalms. Why is all of this in the Bible; could it be for us to see that we are never alone, there were many before us who walked the darkness as well. Spend time reading and seeing that even in Biblical time there were great grievances. God never turned away from a sincere and heartfelt cry and He certainly will not turn away from yours.

O Lord, my God of my salvation,

I cry out day and night before you.

Let my prayer come before you;

incline your ear to my cry!

For my soul is full of troubles,

and my life draws near to Sheol.

I am counted among those who go down to the pit;

I am a man who has no strength,

like one set loose among the dead,

like the slain that lie in the grave,

like those whom you remember no more,

for they are cut off from your hand.

You have put me in the depths of the pit,

in the regions dark and deep.

Your wrath lies heavy upon me,

and you overwhelm me with all your waves. Selah

You have caused my companions to shun me;

you have made me a horror to them.

I am shut in so that I cannot escape;

my eye grows dim through sorrow.
Every day I call upon you, O Lord;
I spread out my hands to you.
Do you work wonders for the dead?
Do the departed rise up to praise you? Selah
Is your steadfast love declared in the grave,
or your faithfulness in Abaddon?
Are your wonders known in the darkness,
or your righteousness in the land of forgetfulness?
But I, O Lord, cry to you;
in the morning my prayer comes before you.
O Lord, why do you cast my soul away?
Why do you hide your face from me?
Afflicted and close to death from my youth up,
I suffer your terrors; I am helpless.
Your wrath has swept over me;
your dreadful assaults destroy me.
They surround me like a flood all day long;
they close in on me together.
You have caused my beloved and my friend to shun me;

my companions have become darkness.

Psalm 88 (ESV)

Take note to where this Psalm ends. It ends with the honest brokenness of one who has also walked such painful darkness. It is not simply one verse, it is indeed several. How we can understand and even greater, how our God can not only understand but desires to relate to us right where we are at. No more pretending, no more putting on a face; we can come just as we are and He will graciously meet us right there. Then, like Footprints in the Sand, He can help carry us to where we need to be.

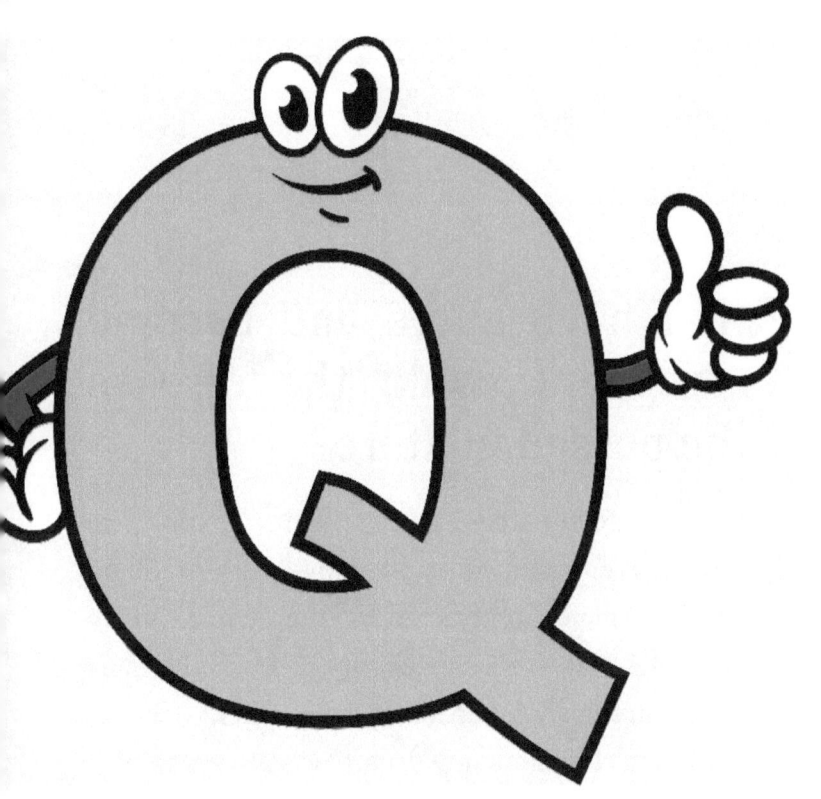

#2

If I have Lyme and become pregnant could the disease be passed in utero?

Unfortunately, yes, Lyme can be transferred from Mom to baby in utero. Some babies have contracted Lyme while being breastfed as well. As children, we sometimes have dreams of becoming NBA stars, Doctors, Fireman, Teachers; my dream was always to be a Mom. I used to write letters to my children; even naming my future daughter, "Summer" as I thought that was the coolest name ever.

I later found those letters and needed to shred most of them as my advice on parenting at age 12 was simply outrageous and there was no way I was allowing such absurdity into my children's hands. Let's see, I believe my early wisdom said kids should pick their curfew and do whatever they want. My absolute passion in life, from that early age, was motherhood. Again, I went through life just thinking that was a given. I wanted kids so I would have them.

I became pregnant at age 22 with our first child. Lani was born a healthy beautiful baby girl. Luke followed two years later born four weeks early weighing in at 7lbs 14oz. I love remembering the RN on duty in the hallway, "Did you see that baby boy born four weeks early at 7lbs. 14oz?" We were told Luke would have to stay in the NICU for a few weeks, I remember being devastated by that news only to hear 48 hours later, "He's doing really well, you can take him home with you." Shaun, our last baby, was born nearly two years later in 2007. Again, blessed with a healthy baby and yet, in 2007, that is when my symptoms of Lyme began.

When I realized the dates involved in my diagnosis, I began to wonder if Lyme had any effect on Shaun. I called my Natural Doctor turned friend and said I wanted to check all three of my children for Lyme. Through muscle testing, we started with Lani and she was clear of Lyme. Luke, too, was clear of Lyme. Shaun's turn came up and I felt anxious as I did breastfeed all three of my children and he was born the same year, I was stricken with Lyme. Shaun's system did recognize Lyme and I held it together as I felt so many emotions begin to creep up; I did not want my son in any way to worry.

I began to pray and ask God to please take any little implication of Lyme in Shaun and give it to me. I was fighting already why would my son have to fight as well? I spent years lamenting this news; I spent years feeling guilty as if I did this to my son. Many Moms have had to deal with such emotion and even on a larger scale than I ever had to. Breastfeeding is a beautiful experience. There's a connection that is stunning between Mom and infant during these times. I truly believe and know that through Lyme life, Satan seeks to demolish and destroy any and all things beautiful.

I fell for the guilt trips and I succumbed several times to the tainting of experiences that were gifts from God. I broke so many times from believing the lies I was told. Shaun is a healthy and joyful spirit and I am happy to proclaim him healed and well. I believe his system recognized Lyme because we were connected at that time yet, through prayer, through believing the absolute power of God to heal, Shaun's body does not recognize Lyme anymore. I know as Mother's we want to keep our children as safe as possible. I know we hold ourselves to a very high standard.

Ok, maybe not all mothers, but I would like to believe most of us want only the very best for our children. This news of Lyme and how it can be passed is hard to cope with yet, we must. We did not ask for Lyme. We truly can become our very worst enemy when we place so much blame on ourselves. Sadly, and again with a heavy heart, miscarriages are very real in our Lyme family. I look back at my ignorant self, early on dreaming of having children and just believing that was what happened for anyone wanting a family. Because my longing was so great and understanding Lyme steals and destroys, my heart is so heavy for all those who have lost their children, whether in utero or stillborn. This is when I am almost tempted to hate Lyme. My hatred begins to flare when I think of a Mother needing to say goodbye to her baby, to her child. I simply want to hold all those mothers in my arms and weep right along with you.

I know it would seem insensitive to ask any Mother who has lost their baby to Lyme a question, but I have to, could you please not blame yourself? Lyme mimics, it loves to hide and seek permanent destruction, it will try its hardest to take down any and all hosts; Lyme is an intruder and therefore, trespasses and invades. We would never wish that on our children as we never wished it upon ourselves. We are not to blame; we are not guilty as charged. We were, too, invaded.

Please forgive yourself and find peace by allowing yourself to grieve and lament as needed. I used to walk around the house, that is my Aunt's or Parent's as we lived with them for a time, and say, "Get it out!" Sometimes we need to go to God and just be a mess. I remember a small group leader several years back as I sat down angry and tried to share where I was in life only to hear, "Don't you talk about my God like that!" Actually, we need to be allowing one another to hurt, grieve, question, and even be confused. We need to address these emotions and feelings otherwise, we are simply pushing them aside and putting on a face.

Where is healing found in ignoring pain? We cannot and will not heal if we won't first allow ourselves and others to walk the hurt. Jesus went to the Father in this way; so what is the Bible showing us? If Jesus went to the Father in that garden and asked why, then we too, can trust God with our why groaning as well. Why would we stop our loved ones from grieving when Jesus grieved as well? If we are not trusting God with our pain and being genuine in our prayer, then are we not simply trying to achieve His love and grace? We do not need to achieve or to be or to do; we simply need to come to Him as we are.

It is through my darkest most real cries, screams, carpet staining sobs that I could get to know my Father's love. C.S. Lewis put it this way, God doesn't want something from us, He simply wants us.

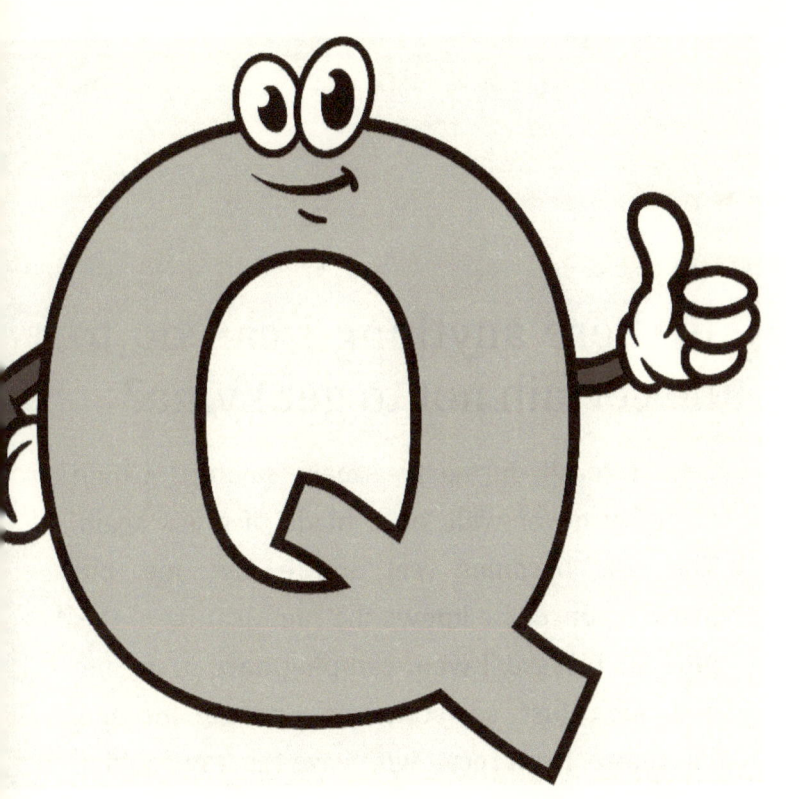

#3

Is there anything I can do to be certain not to get Lyme?

I recall during treatment saying I would basically never walk on a blade of grass again. The fear becomes real and excuse me, but justified, once one knows the ramification of this hideous disease. I went camping once in my life and let's just say once is enough for me. Therefore, I can recall with ease the day, looking back seven years prior to diagnosis, I contracted Lyme. We took a little hike as a family; there I was walking around the trail clueless in flip-flops.

Was it smart to hike in flip flops? No. Did I have a clue what ticks were capable of? No. I have since walked a tiny trail in the neighborhood and yes, I do take precaution, however, I did choose to walk it. There is a line, I believe, between being overly cautious and somewhat aloof. I took on that trail and stayed in the middle and I do not allow my dog to roam free in any high grass or forest preserve areas.

Some may say, hiking is fine if you wear light colored clothing, long socks, and pants tucked into your socks, long sleeves and do a tick check immediately following. Again, up to the individual and their own passion for the outdoors; simply put, if you want to go for a hike, do not do as I did and wear your beach attire. In any and all areas in life, it is good to be knowledgeable and proceed wisely. I should admit, the trail I walked was about 30-40 feet and cemented through that forest area. There is always the question, "Do you think the Lord gave you Lyme disease for a reason?"

First of all, I have no idea what the Lord is up to; the plan He has set for my life. I could not draw it up or design it myself if I tried. I am sitting here at 39 years old and have no clue where my life is headed. I do know, if I am still here and still breathing then He is not finished with me yet. I do not believe the Lord "Gave" me Lyme disease; we do know, however, He allowed it. Like Job, God did not "Do" all of that to Job; He allowed it. Satan was able, by the Lord's admittance, to attack Job yet not take his life.

Job went through so much loss and pain. He endured every blow from Evil and yet, as in Genesis 50, what the Devil meant for harm, the Lord will use for good. Lyme disease attacked my life, my being, my family, my finances, my memory, and much more. This happened. Now, the challenge is live life not focusing on what Lyme has taken away but what I have gained because of it. My marriage fell apart and I had moved in with family along with our children. We arrived at my Aunt's home in June 2014. The children just learned they would be moving and their parents were going to be going through a divorce; I did not want them to start in a new school district on top of all of that. I decided to homeschool them. What was I thinking?!

I say that with a smile on my face because I had just started treatment and was very low on the scale of ability but sure let's teach sixth, fourth, and first grade. God knew. God saw the need and blessing of spending that year together. We all need time; time to stop and just talk. Stop and allow one or all of us to just cry. The children needed to be heard and have their concerns addressed.

I still remember teaching Shaun synonyms and asking that first question, "What is a synonym for food?" I was expecting as we just addressed synonyms, I would hear burger or fries but no, my six year old responded, "Entrée." Thank God I was homeschooling him at first-grade level! Lani was upset as I had to grade her first paper and through my grading chart, she deserved an F. Try being "Mom" turned "Teacher" handing over an F. Oh the waterworks but let me just say, Lani's writing today is beautifully done. No, I am not saying I forever changed my daughter's writing ability; I am saying what a blessing to have had that year with her to work through all things personal plus educational.

Luke's writing went from one sentence to paragraphs, he was so interested in our books that we would read as a family together and when he would get frustrated or down on himself, I was able to simply be there to push him to know what he was capable of. Those three children amazed me daily with their perseverance. I loved working on our Christmas Concert together and lost it, I mean lost it sobbing when they sang that Concert for family. Their puppet show, all handmade, beautiful creations; I still watch that video and smile.

I didn't smile much for years and yet, when I did, there were usually one, two, or three reasons; the day to day little moments with Lani, Luke, and Shaun. In many ways, they kept me going for just one more day. They were the artists behind "Lyme One Day at a Time" as we decided in my parent's basement that day to publish a book together. They were so excited at the thought of being published at a young age. We sat there together for several hours at a time. They all worked hard on their artwork for the book, and then we got the call that we would have to do all the artwork again as our pages would not fit the book template. This was a blow to all of us. In fact, I told them to give me a few minutes to cry and then we would talk about it.

After feeling sorry for myself, I spoke with the three of them and talked about how hard they had worked, and all the hours spent getting those pages ready only to find out they'd have to start all over again. I told them if they didn't want to go through that again; they did not have to. Without hesitation, all three wanted to go for it again. Again, I was amazed by these three, such perseverance. We all sat at that table for the next two days straight completing each and every little detail to those drawings.

Our book was published; we did that together. Why am I telling you all of this when the question was, "Is there anything I can do to be certain not to get Lyme?" Lyme happens. We can be wise in our decisions concerning the outdoors, hikes, tick checks, and our pets but can we be absolutely certain, no. Ticks can be in our grass, I saw one on our kitchen countertop in our

TN house, my son had one on his hip in the shower, and I found one in my bra. These occurrences happened after I contracted Lyme already. However, just because I have lived with Lyme this does not mean I have not been blessed because of it or through it.

I am in no way minimizing the pain and agony it presents but I will continue to shed light on the blessings along the way. After all, this is how we survive. We see victory in the puppet shows our kids perform, the strength it teaches our families (many times without even knowing it), the greater compassion we begin to possess. It is through Lyme that I found hope. That sounds ridiculous and yet it is true.

Prior to the biggest trial in my life, I simply went day to day with a false sense of security. I had my abilities which I treated like normalcy over privilege and lived life accordingly. I got up. Took care of the kids. Took care of the house. Went along as I pleased. Clueless, to any sense of hope because I simply depended on myself and it seemed to be going okay enough. Okay, enough?!

God does not want, "Okay enough," for His children! God wants the very best for us and sometimes that means bringing us down to our knees to first, find Him.

I walked around saying I had faith; it is easy to say I have faith when I did not have anything testing that. It is through fire that our faith is tested and only then do we find a need for the very faith we proclaim. Look what the Lord did for Job. We see at the end of Job, not only does the Lord restore yet He blesses Job's life more so in his latter days. The battle will not be easy yet, in time, the Lord can turn our mess into something grand and beautiful. Picture a bunch of puzzle pieces thrown about; all we see is a mess but in time, what we do not yet see, will turn into a beautiful picture or plan for our life. So whether it's cancer, Lyme, MS, RA, ALS, whatever it may be; we may never be certain we will not face the hardship but we can be certain not to face it alone.

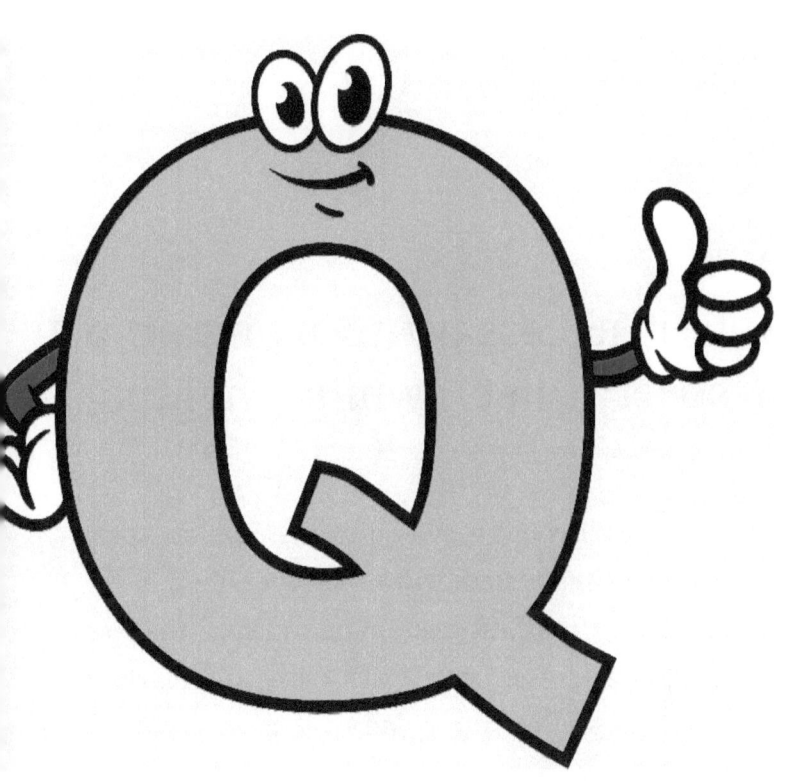

#4

Is it necessary to maintain a strict diet while fighting Lyme?

Yes. I could move on to the next question because simply stated, yes. However, diet, in my opinion, is the first step or first change that we need to address. Lyme loves dairy, therefore, if we cheat and consume dairy we are feeding the very enemy we wish to destroy. Some have cheated and then paid for it in the coming days, seeing an increase in their symptoms. Is it hard to let go of our favorite foods, drinks, treats, etc.? Of course it is. I still remember the Doctor saying over the phone, "No dairy, no gluten, no alcohol, no soy, no sugar, and as organic as possible." There isn't a simple switch, yet, there is a simple choice. Do I stop all this immediately? Yes. Will I figure this all out immediately? No. It's a process to find the best brands and best options; I remember being shocked actually reading through the labels in our pantry.

I had no idea sugar made its way into so many food options. I also spent several hours researching names on labels only to find just how artificial something claiming to be natural was. I once bought an "All natural" product and brought it into our home trusting those two words to be true while turning that jar around and seeing yellow 5, which is artificial food coloring! We are our first line of defense for our bodies; it is crucial what we put in as it will either help or hurt our fight.

Through my treatment years, I had to eliminate some foods for a time, which always interested me. I would eat egg and then I noticed eggs would make me nauseous. These symptoms with food happened often and I chose to listen and trust my body. I noticed this with bananas as well; but now my body is loving bananas. The most interesting, to me, was one month straight I craved celery; I needed it like I needed my next breath. I am not the biggest celery fan at all, again, why we need to listen to our bodies; my body must have needed certain nutrients found in that celery. I can say in all honesty, if you do not give your body the proper nutrition in this battle; you will not win. We cannot stay in a mode of feeling sorry for ourselves for too long either.

I have grown used to the diet I am on and do not intend to change it anytime soon. Yes, it can be awkward when we are invited to someone's home for dinner or attend a party where they are serving food. I have learned to simply eat before I go and it's kind of a joke in my family that Mom always has her water and nutrition bar with her! As I have gotten older, it has become easier to simply let people know beforehand that my diet is pretty strict due to medical necessity. You'll be surprised, or at least I was, how understanding people can be. If Lyme loves anything, we should be beyond fired up to starve the enemy. Sugar itself suppresses our immune system; we are desperate to gain victory in the opposite direction! We want to help strengthen our immune system for the battle ahead. Just say no to sugar!

Dairy is an inflammatory, in fact, a majority of people have issues digesting dairy. Just say no to dairy! Gluten, again most cannot digest and it too is inflammatory. Just say no to gluten! So then, what are we supposed to eat? In my research, while enduring treatment the opinions were overwhelming, to say the least. I found paleo, ketogenic, absolutely no coffee, coffee is okay, vegetables, only vegetables that are fully cooked, rice, no rice, etc. I could go on and on, point being; the massive overload of information can become daunting.

Best, in my opinion? No two cases are alike; we all experience different symptoms, different co-infections, different circumstances in our lives that certainly affect our healing road. We are truly our best supporter of our body's ability to win the fight against Lyme. We need to listen to our bodies. The ketogenic diet may be the answer for you; it was not for me. Paleo may be the best for some and not others. Many with

Lyme grow frustrated because they read, "This saved me from Lyme," then we all try it ourselves and it does nothing. Let's see, true story here, I recall reading that a woman was healed from her Lyme by a bee sting.

It was a lovely summer day, the sun was out and the birds were chirping. I opened up that back door and headed to that deck in search of the answer. I was going to get stung by a bee that day and sing victory praises loud enough for all the neighbors to join in! I saw him; there he was, my answer. Ok, Lord, I prayed out loud, if this little guy can sting me and take away all of my pain, then Lord Jesus let it be! Ok, that bee flew away that very second. I would put my arms out on a hot day walking past their hive, I would stay in that garage when that little one just would not leave and wouldn't you know, both of my sons were stung instead that summer!

God bless anyone who found the answer in the hive; it was not my healing answer to have. That is one example of how desperate we all can become to have our healing right now! I tried everything from medication, IV therapies, Vitamin C, Glutathione, UV, several vitamins, drops, essential oils, healing prayer with oil, Epsom salt baths, body brushing, detox massage, daily organic lemon water, four-month PICC line treatment, and had to decline other treatments suggested such as hyperbaric oxygen therapy due to financial ruin. What do I believe helped me from that list? I believe there was a purpose in all of it.

Being a proponent of all things natural, it was devastating to be on so many medications and inserting PICC line treatment twice daily for four months. Some say all natural is the only way to go with Lyme; believe me when I say all natural is my way of life so I could easily just agree with this statement. However, and again, it is essential that we realize my Lyme fight was mine. Having Lyme for seven years without a diagnosis, it had a field day within me.

Find your team and surround yourself with those who have the same goal in mind; beat Lyme, one day at a time! I trusted everyone from my M.D. at the beginning of the fight who gave me the gift of diagnosis and immediate treatment plan to my Natural Dr. throughout the fight who both encouraged me and at times challenged me to keep pushing forward through the pain. I trusted my IV Dr. with all suggestion resulting from extensive bloodwork and my detox massage therapist who helped ensure the body's willingness to be well. Regardless of who or what or when or how; the important thing is that we, as individuals in this battle, support and encourage one another in our own journey to victory. Again, so many have lost the battle by way of suicide and to have had one of us sitting by their side; a voice to simply agree that this journey is long and hard but to keep pushing until you find your answer.

My answer did not come in a beautifully wrapped package containing one simple gift; my answer was in every little-defined detail in this fight. We need to claim victory before we see it, truly, as our body is fighting and is doing something; we may not be able to necessarily feel our body winning, in fact, we may feel like our body is losing, yet, there is victory in the killing of Lyme and the detox process. Again, these paths along the way may not feel victorious and yet they are. Reminding ourselves, like faith, we cannot see, yet, we can choose to believe.

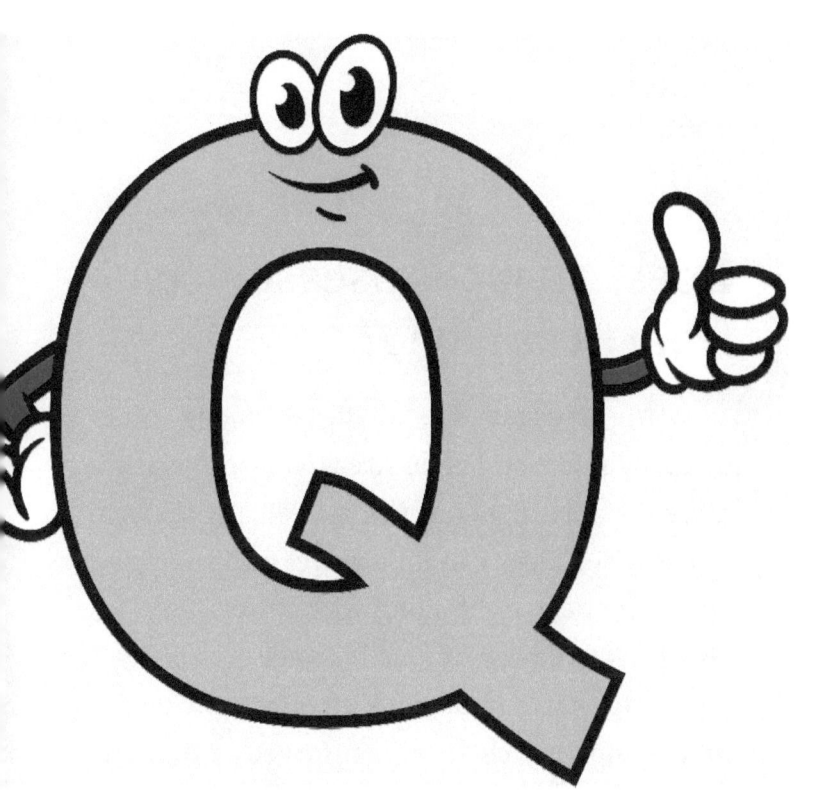

#5

Does Lyme disease come from ticks alone?

No. Mosquitos and fleas among other insects can cause Lyme. Areas where there are more deer are higher at risk as well as ticks tend to love deer. Deer can then travel into your yard and bring ticks right along with them. Ticks can also travel indoors on our beloved pets as well. Yes, I have had to pull a tick off our dog. That is a time I hope my children can forget as I was so angry seeing that tick embedded. I had a surge of emotions as I was fighting Lyme myself, why then did I have to see that nasty tick in my beloved pet? Understand, it is not as if we went for a hike with our dog. We were simply at a park. That tick was hanging out in the grass.

I think that is why I was so upset; you try to do your best to protect and make wise decisions; I was not concerned that day in regard to the lawn my family was nearby. Scary to think, ticks are in the grass. There is a lot of focus on forest, fields, and high grasslands but ticks live in grass as well. Think about it this way, ticks need to eat or feed too so they will do what they have to look for a host. I do not mean to frighten and again, simply being aware of our surroundings and maintaining precaution can go a long way in preventing Lyme.

What do we do when we find a tick embedded? I covered my hand that day with a glove and used a tweezer to get as near to my dog's skin as possible where that tick was embedded. Once I felt like I had a good position, I grabbed and began to pull directly upward. It is necessary to give steady pressure as you pull upward. Once removed, I placed the tick in a baggie and no I did not send in for testing because truth be told, I was furious. I went outside and lost it on that baggie, to say the least. Before I had my moment with that baggie, I rubbed the area on our dog with an alcohol wipe.

Now, there is an option if we find ourselves in a situation like this, to send in the tick for testing. There are Laboratories that can help determine if the tick carries disease organisms. When my family was living in Tennessee, I recall that day when I heard our son Luke from upstairs, "Mom, can you come here?" I made my way upstairs and Luke had just come in from outside and took a shower, "There's something on my privates." I looked and there it was; a tick was embedded in my son. The good thing was, I had optimism that this just occurred as he just came in from outside. In my mind, I wanted to simply cry at this point. We acted quickly and by God's grace, my son lived through that bite with no symptom whatsoever. I choose not to send in that tick as we responded immediately, and I had a trusted Natural Dr. to go to for advice and counsel at any time.

I was so proud of my son that he took notice and asked for help. Many do not see the tick; he did not see it himself he felt something on him during his shower. Thank God he spoke up. There is a possibility any one of us can become a tick's target; if we see a tick embedded, we do not need to panic. Not all ticks carry Lyme and if we respond as soon as possible, our chance at deflection is much higher. I was angry when I saw that tick on our dog and I felt completely broken when I saw that tick on my son. Our emotions can run high, our tears can flow, and we can be truly tested when here we are fighting Lyme life and we see a tick attack a loved one. Yes, it is a possibility and yes, ticks are everywhere. However, yes, we can remember that we have the power to be aware of and if necessary, to act immediately.

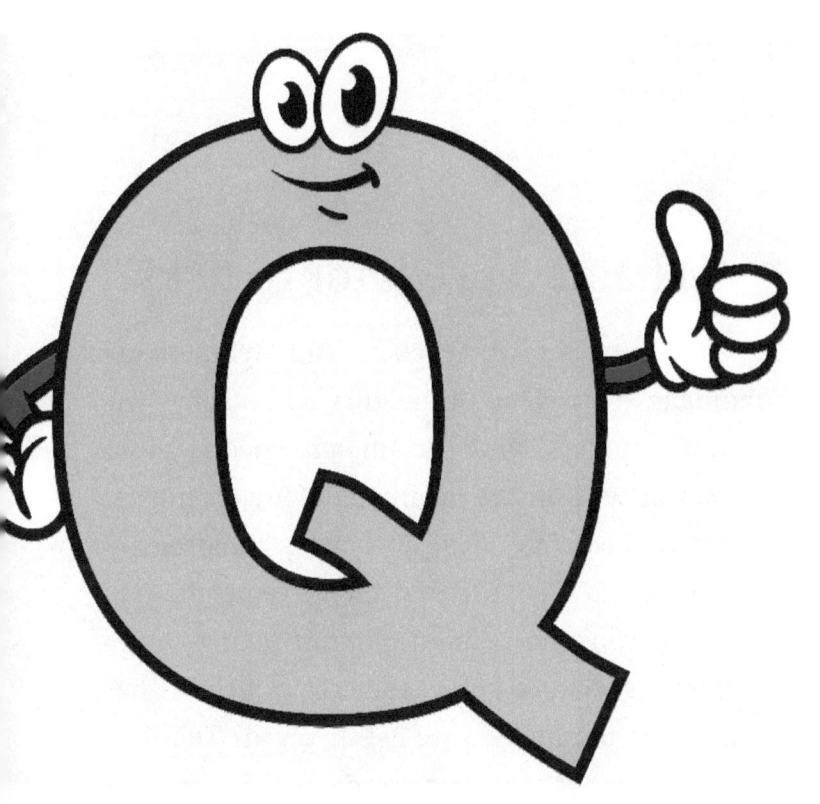

#6

What is a predator to ticks?

Guinea fowl, chicken, and opossum are among the top tick predators while some wild birds, spiders, and certain ant species attack ticks as well. At the beginning of my diagnosis, I entertained the idea of having hundreds of chickens in our yard and then I remembered, I didn't want the responsibility of taking care of chickens! Nature helps take care of ticks as best as it can but how do we get involved? There are certain things we can do to deter ticks from our yards.

It is a good idea to first clean up our yards as best we can, mowing often, removing any and all leaf piles, and clearing any tall grasslands or reeds from our properties. Ticks are attracted to Japanese Barberry plants, so removal is crucial if found on your property as well. On the flip side, there are plants to deter ticks as well. Ticks do not like lavender, garlic, sage, mint, lemongrass, and rosemary plants, to name a few. Ticks do not prefer direct sun exposure, they like moist and humid environments. Which as a parent, we tend to want to place our children's playsets, sandboxes, trampolines, etc in the shade. I know we did!

However, it is better to lower the risk by placing such items in the sun; just tell the children to wear hats and use sunscreen. Ticks enjoy a simple way of travel and do not appreciate any rocky surfaces, therefore, another way to decrease tick population in our yards is to place a border between the yard and any grassy fields or wooded area. It is best to use gravel or dry wood chips to place about a three-foot border. Another natural approach to deterring ticks from our property is the use of essential oils. I use water, witch hazel, with a combination of different essential oils. I have used lavender, lemongrass, eucalyptus, rosemary lemon, and peppermint essential oil. This can also be sprayed topically on our lawns as well. I tend to use this natural approach with my family as a preferred spray and our dog as well.

In addition to the spray, I like to place a few drops of essential oil on shoes as well. Both my daughter and my one son went on a camping trip with their school. My internal reaction to this news was mixed, to say the least. I wanted them to go and gain new experiences, but I was aware of the very real possibility they would be near a higher tick population. We spoke about the possibility and I did send them with spray and treated their shoes as well.

I know DEET is brought up as a means to deter ticks. Again, personal preference, however, I just want to caution using any chemicals on our skin directly or our lawn where young children can come into contact with it. Some choose to treat only clothing and shoes with DEET without spraying topically. Diatomaceous Earth or DE is a good option to use and it is multi-faceted, which is a bonus! Spread, as it is like a powder, around areas in your yard that have more foliage or near areas where any animal may be hiding out. It is a good idea to also do a dusting around the foundation of your home as well. DE can be dusted onto our pet's fur and skin safely as well.

I know there is so much information out there now and again this can become overwhelming. The goal is simply to have as much knowledge as possible and then decide what will work best for your home and family. We all can agree on one thing, we do not want to give ticks an opportunity to call our home their own.

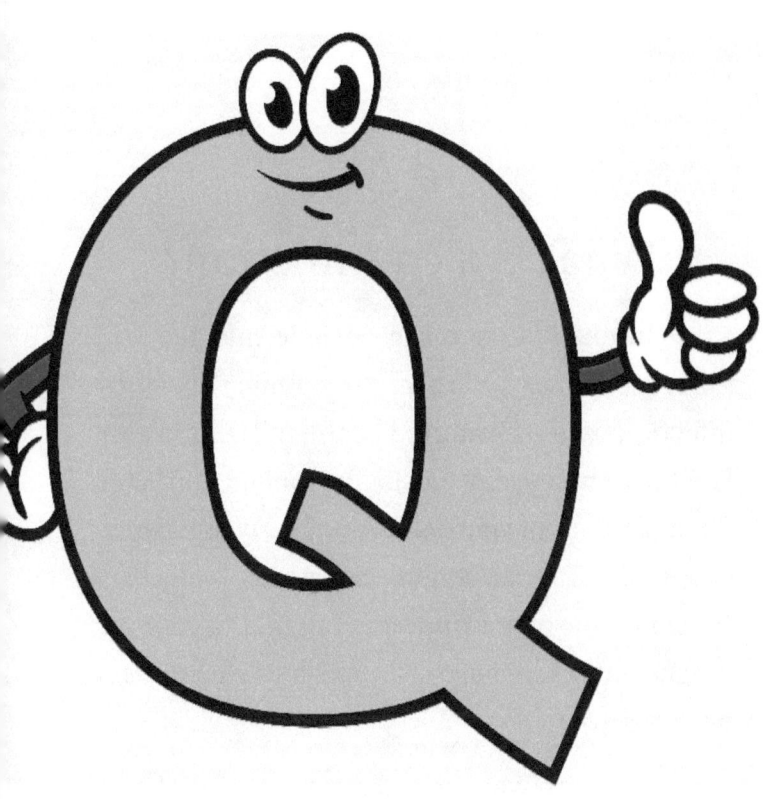

#7

#7
What is a co-infection?

In one bite, one can become infected with different bacteria, viruses, and fungi. These co-infections are transmitted at the initial infection. Most common are, Babesia, Bartonella, Ehrlichia, Rocky Mountain spotted fever and Mycoplasma. I had each of these among others as well. Each causing their own symptoms ranging from fever, fatigue, muscle ache, chest pain, and shortness of breath.

When I was first diagnosed with Lyme, Babesia, Borrelia, and C. Pneumonia were all present. I found success attacking co-infections with different products from the Pure Formulas Series Kits to DesBio products identifying specific viruses. As one virus seemed to be conquered, another would surface. For lack of a better visual, like an onion, this process is one layer at a time; certain infections would persist more than others and when I saw my Natural Doctor reach for that "Black box," I wanted to just scream, "Another one!"

My symptoms were a wide range; however, I did have neuro Lyme which caused, in my opinion, the most difficult symptoms to face. My memory loss was something I could not explain as I was not diagnosed for seven years. I was riding in the car with my Mom and Aunt in the front seats. They started to talk about a Josh Grobin concert when I chimed in, "Wish I could have gone to a Josh Grobin concert." They simultaneously and slowly began to look at each other. Apparently, I was with them when we went to see Josh Grobin.

Now, we didn't see the concert that night as there was a tiny note on the door that the concert was canceled, yet, I did not remember any of those details. This began to happen often when a family member, friend or sadly my children would ask, "Do you remember...." And I would have to reply, "No." Sometimes I couldn't even respond, especially to my children asking me if I had a memory about a birthday party or event; those memories were stolen away.

I spent a long time feeling sorry for myself in regard to lost precious memories. I had to tell myself, over time, countless people suffer dementia sadly and numerous have lost their precious photos and memorabilia to house fires. It is so crucial during the Lyme life fight to give ourselves an opportunity to mourn while reminding ourselves to search for the positive. Positive? What could be positive while losing memory, struggling to breathe, not remembering a word in the middle of your sentence, not understanding why your heart is beating as if you just ran a marathon even though you're lying in bed? Where's the positive in that? It's not in that, no, but it is nearby.

For me, it was the blue jays that God placed right outside our home in Tennessee for the entire month of January. I sat there alone, and suffering greatly and yet, when I would look outside there they were, just for me, a reminder that God was in this with me. It was in the random cards that would come in the mail to me with words of encouragement and prayer, sometimes, from people I had never met. It was there when I had to sell my car for money. There I was a mom of three with no way of getting around and then I opened that card from my Grandmother to find, "Here's $5,000, please find a car for your family."

I am positive we all have things that mean something to us; it is unexplainable; therefore, it is our Heavenly Father. I am sure of this; I see rays of the sunshine poking through the clouds and it just means something to me. The Lord, if you are willing to see, tries to communicate with you through his beautiful creation. The Lord places people in our path at the right time; sometimes at the right second. My newest attempt to fight the urge to be negative is to respond to any and all pouting, muttering, or complaining by saying, "I'm grateful." That's it. Two little words to get my brain back on track. Co-infections have landed me in the ER and allow me to say, what a waste of time and money! How many times, I had to look into a Doctor's puzzling glare. I would start communication promptly about Lyme and literally some Doctor's never came within a foot of me! One actually stood in the doorway and simply shrugged while ordering pointless tests. Stupid me to take so long figuring out that they were incapable of helping me!

Yeah, I said it. I can say that on top of any rooftop on any day because that was my personal experience. Truthfully, the Doctor I admired the most, on one of my several ER trips, looked at me after Lyme was mentioned and honestly said, "We cannot help you here." Exactly! Co-infection communication needs to improve in the medical world and I am very happy to see Lyme being taken more and more seriously.

Now, we need to see movement, education for the medical world, accurate treatments when needed, and how about insurance starts covering all costs? How frustrated I would become when I knew co-infections were causing great pain, like the pain in my lungs or my right kidney, and no one could help. There I was explaining Lyme disease, in need of something to help the pain subside, and all I received was the blank stares, the exit slip, or hundreds of dollars spent on pointless tests. I had seizure activity startup and again, as I was not diagnosed for seven years, I spent a lot of time in the Neuro world. I would pass all the tests and one Dr. actually put his hands in the air and shrugged, "I don't know, MS?" I looked at him and said, "Are you asking me?!"

That was a quick exit and a joy to receive, still, a bill of service. Co-infections are a very real threat with Lyme. Each co-infection requires specific treatment relating to its own tendencies. This battle can be won; wars can last several years and in many ways fighting co-infections is like fighting in a war. You may have sweet victory over one enemy or infection only to face something hiding around the corner. Where's the end? There's no end; there's right now, today. Do what you can with today and let tomorrow come as it may.

I recall my Lyme MD saying treatment would be two years; two years passed, and I was still suffering. I remember that was hard as I would cry, "But it's been the two years Lord!?" If we do not put the pressure on our body to have a specified end date, our battle will be more victorious fighting day by day! Trust me, do not look to a year from now; if you beat one co-infection; you're a winner. You now know your body is getting stronger; remember I did not say feel stronger. The proof is in the day to day victories. I may still lose my breath quicker than I would like but I no longer struggle to breathe. I may feel my heart race with little exercise but my heart no longer races while I am simply lying in bed. I may not be where I would like in my overall healing, but I sure am not where I was years ago.

My breathing didn't change in a day nor did my cardiac symptoms but that doesn't mean the fight wasn't being won daily. I encourage you during the co-infection fights you will face to drink organic lemon water daily. This seemed to help my body detox best. Again, maybe your system will respond better to Epsom salt baths or body brushing, whatever the case may be, may you find exactly what works best for your body! You have to understand some of our sickest days, excuse me, but days spent on the toilet are actually very victorious; our body is eliminating at its best! It doesn't feel like our best day, but it is movement in the right direction!

When I first started treatment for Lyme, I was unable to sleep well at all. This affected the journey greatly; I would still try to be lights out by 10p.m. and up at 7a.m. Trying to train our bodies and get them on a sleep schedule; over time, now my body is sleeping much better than before. Be kind to yourself and if that's too hard, be kind to your body. What?! Yes, this helped me tremendously. To myself, I was a failure in many ways. I was in my mid-thirties living with family, nearly divorced, and unable to do pretty much anything. The temptation while facing the fight of the co-infections was to label myself a loser daily. Yet, here my body was facing this uphill battle and I was the only one who could help it out; my body didn't ask for this!

I would tap those legs and encourage them to walk one more step or flight of stairs. I would say on occasion, "It's okay body," or even, "I'm sorry," when I had to administer medical treatment. I know this helped me not only to get in a state of mind to fight back but also and over time, with self-esteem. That encouragement to walk one more flight of stairs became a walk down the driveway to today being able to do squats and walk around the block. Over time, and slowly, I began to see my body getting stronger, then I could see that maybe I wasn't a loser; maybe I was stronger than I ever gave myself credit for.

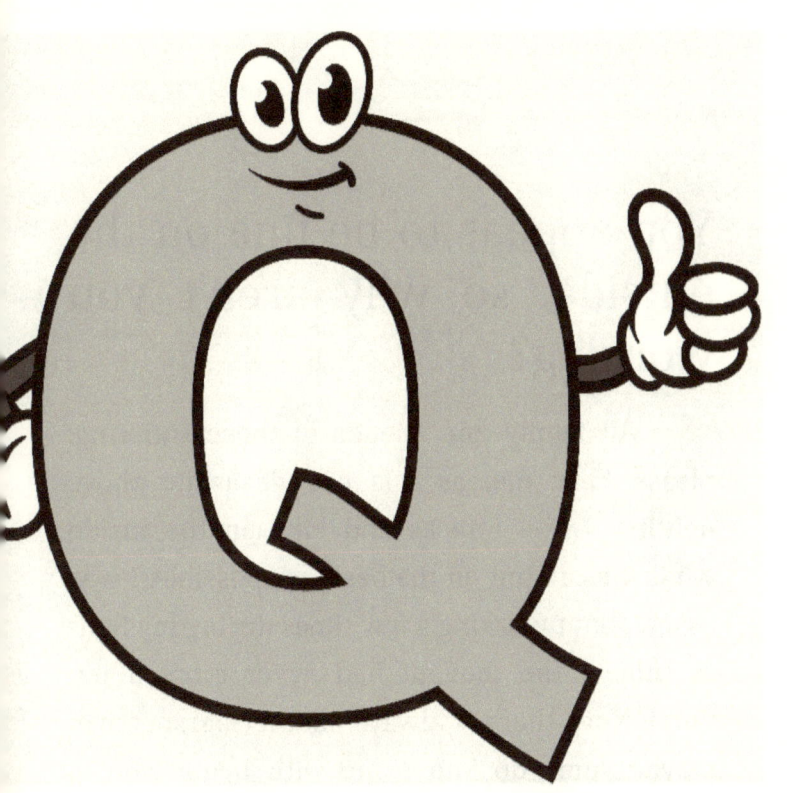

#8

You appear to be fine on the outside, so why aren't you working?

All family and friends of those suffering, please hear me, as this can devastate those fighting. Lyme attacks and kills on the inside while we can put on the best face possible. I was asked about working a few times during my fight as though the thought had never crossed my mind. Now, there is always another perspective; maybe some do know one with Lyme who is choosing to sabotage their fight by not following Doctor's orders or sticking to a very strict plan, diet, and routine. However, those diagnosed late stage or chronic have a very tough battle at hand.

We are not easily pointed out as in the case of those fighting cancer who have lost their hair due to treatment. Does this mean that we are simply ok because we appear to be ok on the outside? No. Similar to those fighting depression; the battleground is not in our immediate appearance, therefore, the quick judgment can be rather painful. I thought about working every single day of my fight and still do. Nobody wanted more for my children then I did as I saw their worried faces each and every time they witnessed their Mom really struggling. Late-stage chronic Lyme is not like a cold or virus that passes in a few weeks; this is a battle physically, mentally, emotionally, and yes, spiritually as well. The one walking the battle lives daily in their mind with many of the same questions friends and family may have. Best to just communicate openly and honestly but please do not simply assume based off appearance.

I had tried a support group in the beginning; whether that helps or not is up to each individual. However, family and friends may need to seek their own support as well, as living the Lyme journey alongside us, can be exhausting for you as well. My family was huge support throughout my Lyme journey. When I was unable to move around much, my family would walk the kids to the bus stop, drive to soccer practices and games, attend school events, etc. Yes, my heart was broken and, in some ways, it still is, at not being able to do basic daily activities with my children for some time, however, I was blessed in that I had family step in and sacrifice their own time and privacy to help us out.

After some time, this can become taxing on anyone. Relationships can become strained, things can be said, and accusations made. Lyme will tear apart families due to its longevity and severity. I believe our divorce stats are close to 95%; I am not shocked by this number in any way. For months we can become bedridden and our bodies can only handle treatment and detox. Then we can have what seems like several good weeks in a row where, if you're like me you start praising that healing hath come upon you, only to find yourself back down in the lonely, depleting, painful grip of Lyme and co-infection.

It's a war, truly, a battle that takes our time, money, energy, and sadly it can kill relationships and most devastatingly, can lead some to choose to end their life. I had been asked about getting a job at the same time as the declaration that I would need help possibly the rest of my life. Please be as uplifting as possible; one with Lyme does not need to hear they'll basically be nobody their whole life; they may already be dealing with that lie in their mind.

Fighting Lyme is a very lonely existence; we are left mainly with ourselves which means our minds are the loudest voice in the room. All the debilitating thoughts we can come into agreement with because our outlook may not appear to be good. We take one thought into an agreement and we invite evil to dictate our thoughts as well. This battle becomes a warzone of the mind. Why aren't you working? How many times I wanted to just scream, "You live Lyme for one day and let me see you head out for interviews!" I wouldn't however, probably by God's grace or pure weakness physically to endure such conversation. Thing is, the battle is thinking behind that comment is something derogatory, such as YOU LOSER! This is how many Lyme warriors slip into depression; feeling like we are not measuring up or we are not useful for anything at all. *You're a loser, Shannon, look at you, your children are going to grow up thinking you were just sickly and broken all the time.*

Truth, my children have grown so strong through this with such compassionate hearts God must have great plans for them! *Shannon, you're going to be sick your whole life and be unable to do anything important.* Truth, I'm not where I was a year or two ago as I am headed toward healing; as it is written, "Heal me, O Lord, and I shall be healed; save me, and I shall be saved: for You are my praise." (Jeremiah 17:14) *Shannon, God doesn't care about you; if God cared about you where is He now?* Truth, as it is written, "...do not fear, for I am with you; do not be dismayed, for I am your God. I will strengthen you and help you; I will uphold you with my righteous right hand." (Isaiah 41:10) Where does that come from, it is written? Jesus Himself was in the desert for 40 days and was tempted by the devil. Jesus in His response would declare, "It is written," along with the power of the Word. Again, to lead us when we too, will combat evil. Evil comes in many forms; it hates and wants to destroy. Our minds must fight this battle daily; with Him all things are possible.

Notice, it never states all things will be pleasant or easy. Yet, all things are possible when we let God take the lead and fight back just as Jesus did. No matter the comments, no matter the thoughts, we do not owe an explanation to anyone who does not wish to understand. Bullying is in the world and sadly it has even caused some to take their own lives. We do not need to accept others' opinions of our Lyme journey, rude comments, or even the lingering looks. We need to draw near to Him who knows our suffering and rebuke any and all attempts to bring us further into darkness.

Like the song from Hillsong "Still," declares, "Hide me now under Your wings, cover me within Your mighty hands... when the oceans rise and thunder roar, I will soar with you above the storm...I will be still and know You are God." We do not need to please others or make them happy; simply rest in His truth of who you are and all you were created to be!

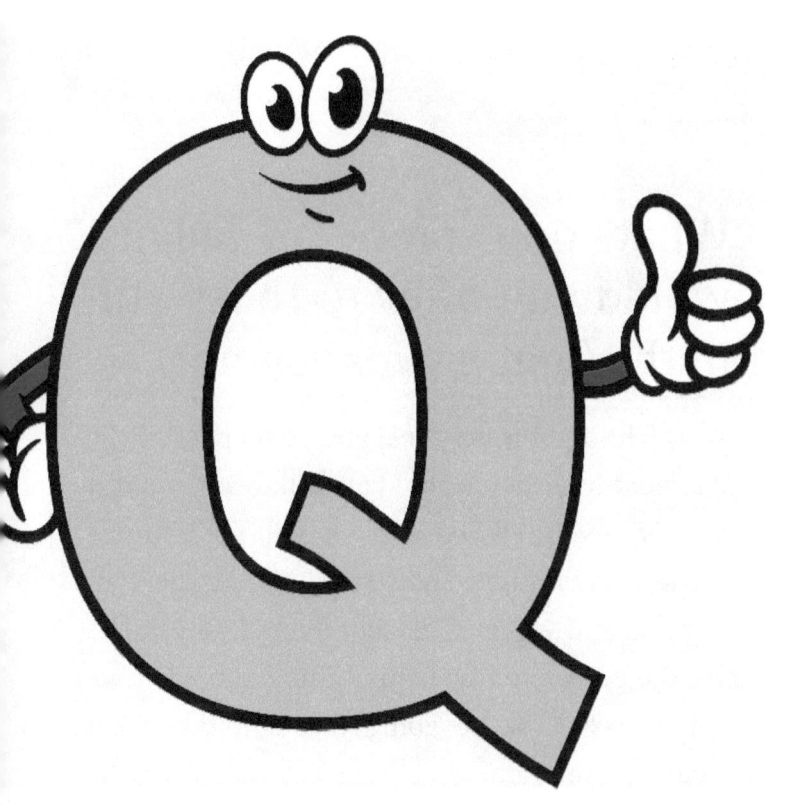

#9

What one piece of advice would you offer to those still in the fight against Lyme?

This fight is very real and could possibly be the most intense journey you will face. To put it bluntly, if you tell yourself you will not win this battle; you will not. The struggle is fifty percent physical and yet, fifty percent mental. Our minds are the power source behind this fight; what we tell ourselves while going through it is what feeds our ability to win. If we focus solely on the damage done, the symptoms, the number of co-infections, without telling ourselves that one day at a time is all we can do and find the simple victory in today; we cannot win if we do not have a winning attitude.

Does that mean, I was singing joyfully and doing victory dances daily? No. Lyme hurts.

Lyme destroys. Lyme steals. That pain and the loss is very real and needs to be addressed, absolutely. I am saying, find victory in today. One of my first goals was to slice pizza. I remember starring down that pizza and my kids needing to eat dinner and I could not do it. I had to accept that today I was not going to slice that pizza but I had to tell my mind and body that while that was ok, we were going to celebrate that first slice I would eventually make! Another goal was walking a staircase. Again, giving my body the support it needed that maybe today it could not do it but there would be a day; I would walk that flight of stairs and we would celebrate! Our body needs us to understand, it needs time to heal while also encouraging it through the fight. While we try to sleep, our bodies never stop trying to locate and destroy the infection. Lyme disease is a one day at a time journey. What you may not be able to do today; there is an opportunity waiting in tomorrow!

I also want to point out the need for forgiveness. Question: if we want to beat Lyme disease, would we be willing to give it our absolute best shot? I would assume we would all declare yes to that one. There is so much pain we stuff deep inside during life that can have a profound effect on our healing. I knew there were people in my life I needed to speak with and some that I needed to forgive. I wanted as much peace over my body and mind as possible; ensuring that my battle with Lyme would not be hindered in any way. I had to take a look back at my childhood, high school, and my college days running from God, all the anger within that seemed to take hold while I even forgot why I was angry in the first place. Who I was and who I had become and where I wanted to be in life. I began to journal again through these times and ask myself questions. Who are you mad at? Why? Some people were easier to let go of and forgive than others.

I was still in the midst of my divorce at this time, when the Lord laid it on my heart to "Stop the divorce." What?! I had grown scared of Chris; I had nothing to say to God on this request besides, "Are you nuts?!" There it was again, "Stop the divorce." I didn't stop the divorce, I decided to be obedient as I wanted to be and put it on a pause. "Wear your wedding ring again." Oh, my Lord Jesus almighty WHAT?! We start to have our adult tantrum which includes many, "But" or "What about when he…" I wanted to convince God, I had a better plan. Yikes.

The first time I forgave Chris, I was lying on the carpet crying and barely able to speak. Well, Chris and I didn't become angelic beings so I put the divorce back on. I figured, well God, I did what you asked kind of and it didn't appear heavenly so I figure you probably want to do things my way now. We kept going through our divorce and I kept fighting the battle one day at a time. "Stop the divorce."

We had been in our divorce process for four years and our end date was fast approaching. Wisdom from a trusted friend, "Shannon, does God ever change His mind?" I was broken, again. All the sudden I had such regret, remorse, and even love toward Chris again. Chris and I stopped the divorce within days of it finishing. I say Chris and me, yet, truly

God is in control. I do not know where life is headed; none of us can declare what tomorrow may bring. Sure, we can plan and fill up our calendars but life just happens. Lyme happened. We can face today; we can win today. Remember, it does not always feel like a win but that does not mean you are not winning.

Win by following a strict diet plan, making a set sleep schedule, detoxing when necessary, finding a trusted medical support team, communicating with family and friends, asking for help, being grateful for the tiniest of privileges you gain back, forgiving hurts from yesterday, moving forward in life, and win by coming back to the One who knows you best and will love you always; come back to the arms of your Heavenly Father. You can win and I believe you will win!

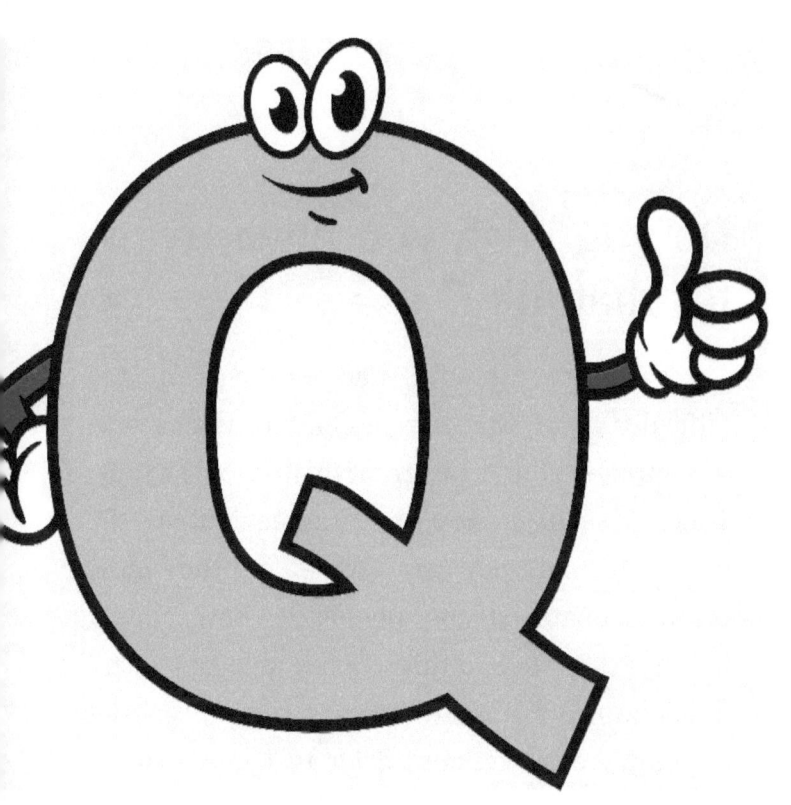

#10

Do you wish you never went for that hike?

Yes and no. If I had any clue of the difficulty ahead that I would endure with Lyme, of course, I would never wish that on anyone. There have been, however, blessings along the way. My children are some of the most compassionate, strong people I know simply because they walked this journey alongside me. I didn't know what it felt like to cry into the carpet in complete brokenness prior to Lyme. I never had to seek the Lord more in all my life.

I have noticed that Lyme broke me down several times and yet, I have begun to heal, and, in its place, there is less judgment; I now walk around and wonder what others have been through or are going through. Simply put, beyond our brokenness and through our healing there can truly be the utmost blessing. Lyme robbed me of time, energy, and memories but Lyme has given me strength I didn't know I had and gratefulness for the little things in life.

Would I rather be walking around as I was prior to this valley? Simply thinking all was okay and okay was good enough I guess. Thinking that life would always be just as it was and oh well. Guessing that maybe I would go to Heaven. Or would I rather be still on the journey, waiting on His promises and knowing that I am loved and never left alone in this life? Knowing that God has given me a gift through the pain; He has opened my heart again and given me hope, of which I never had. I am thankful God has allowed me to find Him in the valley. I guess it does not matter what gets us to find the Lord; regardless, the victory is in my relationship with Him. The victory is in the blessing along the way.

It was a blessing the first time I sliced pizza and it was a blessing when I learned I beat another co-infection. Blessings both big and small are worth praising! Looking back, I would not change going for that hike, however, looking forward, I will never hike in flip-flops again!

Conclusion

2007, walking around that hill, enjoying the day and thinking I was in control of tomorrow. I felt perfectly fine and free, having all abilities right there at my fingertips. Cue the dramatic music and big boom; then my life left me and I was simply alive. Unable to move, breathe, and uncertain of what was taking over me. The emotions, the anger, the frustration, the depression, the darkness; life as I knew it would never be the same. Yet, was that such a bad thing?

Yes, to me it was. I was comfortable where I was. I was used to my life and how it was going. I was in control and perfectly fine with that. Little tiny tick comes along and my world turned upside down. Years of being misunderstood and relationships began to fizzle. The loss was great indeed. What would I possibly gain from this living hell?

What I did gain was humility; truly thinking about others. I gained sympathy for other communities I had not once thought about.

I gained perspective on privilege versus an attitude that being able was simply the norm. I gained an excitement for seeing Jesus Christ's coming! I gained my weak religion turning to a real relationship!

Lyme came to seek, kill, and destroy my life, my marriage, my finances, and yes, my soul. Through healing spiritually, physically, emotionally, and mentally, I would like to thank Lyme. Yes, you read correctly, I would like to thank Lyme for making me stop completely. If I hadn't been broken down and nearly lifeless, I would not have learned what life is truly all about. It is living one day at a time not knowing what tomorrow will bring but trusting that there is a God that will walk this life with you.

Life is not about us (Tough one to learn as I am still learning and will be until my death bed), it is about being loving and kind, patient toward others, having compassion for those less fortunate than ourselves. Our life does not belong to us. We were created for a reason; we are here for a purpose. The fact that I take a next breath is because it is given to me. How are we going to live? Beaten down by Lyme? Yes, it will be hard and yes, it can take a long time to be well; we must fight while we wait.

We are never alone; look at the lady who bled; she waited a long time. Look at Abraham; he waited a long time for his son. Look at David; he waited. Look at the crippled man, the blind, and the lepers! God does not change. He is the very same God yesterday as He is this very day! You keep fighting and if you are reading this and your family member has Lyme; you keep on fighting for them as well!

Don't simply believe you can be well; know you WILL be well and do everything you can to give your body the best day it has had in a long time! Who cares about tomorrow; today you can and will be victorious! Remember, God did not give you Lyme, yes He allowed it but He knows what He can do to turn it ALL for good! That puzzle, it sure is a mess today but when completed; God will reveal its beauty. As a dear counselor used to say to me at each of our goodbyes and now, in her memory, I will pass along in truth to you; you are LOVED.

For Further Study

lymedisease.org - LymeDisease.org is one of the largest non-profit Lyme disease patient advocacy organizations in the world.

ilads.org - The International Lyme and Associated Diseases Society. ILADS is a nonprofit, international, multidisciplinary medical society dedicated to the appropriate diagnosis and treatment of Lyme and associated diseases. Its special mission is to educate medical professionals.

rawlsmd.com – Dr. Bill Rawls is a specialist in treatment for Lyme disease. He is the author of

"*Unlocking Lyme:*

Myths, Truths, and Practical Solutions for

Chronic Lyme Disease"

lymeconnection.org - Lyme Connection represents patients, family members, practitioners, researchers and community members committed to ending the suffering caused by tick-borne diseases. We educate the community about prevention and early diagnosis and support patients.

planetnatural.com/pest-problem-solver/lawn-pests/tick-control/ - There are over 800 species of ticks found worldwide. Here's how to get rid of them in your yard using proven, organic and natural techniques.

About the Author

Shannon Marie has fought Lyme disease and several co-infections for over a decade. Her battle was anything but simple, in fact, many

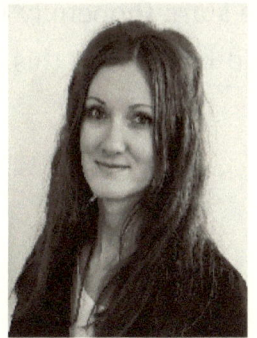

times she got up only to be knocked right back down again. Yet, she was inspired by her children to not give up but instead face one day at a time. Her desire is to help those fighting Lyme to become the warrior they are deep down inside.

Thank you for reading this 10q* book on dealing with Lyme Disease. This would be a great time to post your review in the Kindle store. Follow this link, give it some stars (hopefully five!), and tell us what you liked best about this book. Thanks again.

*10q book - This is an eBook built around ten questions people ask about the topic. 10qaa Publishing is actively seeking authors to write more of these helpful books. For information, please visit http://www.10qaa.com. Remember, it never costs you anything to publish with us. So, now we ask:

"Is there a 10q in you?"

www.ingramcontent.com/pod-product-compliance
Lightning Source LLC
Chambersburg PA
CBHW021847170526
45157CB00007B/2973